BEATING PANIC ATTACKS

5 SIMPLE STEPS TO ELIMINATE PANIC ATTACKS EFFORTLESSLY

EDWARD JONES

Copyright 2019 by Edward Jones - All rights reserved.

This document is geared towards providing exact and reliable information in regards to the topic and issue covered. The publication is sold with the idea that the publisher is not required to render accounting, officially permitted, or otherwise, qualified services. If advice is necessary, legal or professional, a practiced individual in the profession should be ordered.

- From a Declaration of Principles which was accepted and approved equally by a Committee of the American Bar Association and a Committee of Publishers and Associations.

In no way is it legal to reproduce, duplicate, or transmit any part of this document in either electronic means or in printed format. Recording of this publication is strictly prohibited and any storage of this document is not allowed unless with written permission from the publisher. All rights reserved.

The information provided herein is stated to be truthful and consistent, in that any liability, in terms of inattention or otherwise, by any usage or abuse of any policies, processes, or directions contained within is the solitary and utter responsibility of the recipient reader. Under no circumstances will any legal responsibility or blame be held against the publisher for any reparation, damages, or monetary loss due to the information herein, either directly or indirectly.

Respective authors own all copyrights not held by the publisher.

The information herein is offered for informational purposes solely, and is universal as so. The presentation of the information is without contract or any type of guarantee assurance.

The trademarks that are used are without any consent, and the publication of the trademark is without permission or backing by the trademark owner. All trademarks and brands within this book are for clarifying purposes only and are the owned by the owners themselves, not affiliated with this document.

INTRODUCTION

I want to thank you and congratulate you for downloading the book, *Beating Panic Attacks: 5 simple steps to eliminate panic attacks effortlessly.*

This book contains proven steps and strategies on how to completely eliminate panic attacks in 5 simple steps to regain control of your life quickly and easily.

This book also contains a brief overview of panic attacks and panic disorders. It tells you their definitions as well as their common causes and symptoms. Learning about panic attacks and panic disorders can really help you to prepare yourself in case you experience a familiar symptom.

Moreover, this book discusses the five easy techniques and strategies to use if you want to overcome your panic attack quickly and effectively. These steps are about using breathing techniques and meditation to improve your condition so you can regain control of your life.

Thanks again for downloading this book, I hope you enjoy it!

1

WHAT ARE PANIC ATTACKS?

Panic attacks are shitty. Let me just put that out there. If you've ever experienced one, you know what I'm talking about.

The annoying thing is, it's your body just doing its job. It thinks that you're in danger so it kicks in your fight or flight response.

Google defines a panic attack as:

"a sudden feeling of acute and disabling anxiety."

Which seems to sum it up nicely…bummer.

Some people experience panic attacks rarely and others have an on-going struggle with them, sometimes on a daily basis. If that's you, I feel your pain, I feel your struggle and just know, there are many, really simple fixes for it that you can start to implement *today*.

Personally, when I was suffering with these attacks, I had extreme agoraphobia and could barely leave my room. Later on, I had massive anxiety around driving, especially on motorways and would feel an attack coming on if I just thought about having to drive on one.

There's not always a rhyme or reason for why panic attacks happen. Sometimes, like with me and my driving on motorways, it was pretty obvious what would set it off. I had extreme anxiety around a specific situation.

I also had panic attacks out of the blue with no reason whatsoever, in situations I had been in many times before without issue.

I had one at dinner with my better half's family once… that was fun.

According to statistics, at least one in every ten individuals experiences a panic attack at some point. Likewise, at least one in every fifty individuals suffers from panic disorder.

In the US alone, over 60 million people experience panic attacks and over 3 million people suffer from panic disorder —this is how common panic attacks and panic disorder are! So don't worry, you're not alone!

The Signs and Symptoms of Panic Attack

The signs and symptoms of panic attacks tend to show abruptly. They usually reach the peak within a few minutes and may last up to 30 minutes (usually a lot less!) and come sometimes come in waves.

People who experience a panic attack usually find that they experience one or more of the following:

- Dizziness
- Shortness of breath
- Sweating
- Stomachache
- Lightheadedness
- Hyperventilation

- Dry mouth
- Chest pain
- Numbness
- Shaking
- Tingling sensations
- Hot and cold flashes
- Choking feeling
- Fear of losing sanity
- Fear of dying

If you experience a panic attack and you notice any of it's physical symptoms, you may, incorrectly, think you have a physical disorder because of the very real symptoms you experience in the moment. This is not the case. Seriously. You've been through panic attacks before and you're fine right? No heart attacks, you're still sane, no ongoing health issues etc. Likewise, even if you feel that you're really about to die, there is a huge chance that you're actually not.

The symptoms of panic attacks occur prior to you having an overdrive of nervous impulses coming from your brain towards the other parts of your body. So when you have a panic attack, your body may release more hormones, including adrenaline. This prompts you to have a *fight or flight* response.

The fight or flight response is something that is ingrained in your system. It started with our ancestors from the Paleolithic era when they either had to fight the danger in front of them or flee to stay safe and alive. At present, we still experience the fight or flight response whenever we are faced with a dangerous situation, or at least, a situation we perceive as dangerous.

What you might find is that your body may have the same reaction when you experience a panic attack. You may hyperventilate or breathe very heavily. As you do this, you breathe out large amounts of carbon dioxide, causing the acidity of your blood to change. This leads to more symptoms such as cramps, confusion, and sometimes fainting (very rare!).

This imbalance isn't really harmful at all as, once you calm down, the body will naturally balance everything out again. It's basically just a case of breathing slower.

If you recognize yourself in anything you just read, don't worry! There are some fantastic tools and techniques to overcome this and regain control of your life today!

The Causes of Panic Attacks

Experts have not been able to pinpoint any exact cause of panic attack, but they have found that genetics and family history have something to do with it. Those whose family members have panic disorder are also more likely to have it.

In addition, panic attacks can be triggered by exposure to stressful situations like speaking in public or crossing a bridge and even some food and drinks can have an impact as we'll discuss later.

Overcoming Panic Attacks & Panic Disorders

Now, all of that sounds a bit doom and gloom, but fear not! There are some amazing tools and techniques to overcome these issues. Many of which you will find, have an immediate impact, and the others will help you to be more relaxed and happier on an on-going basis.

Let's get to it, shall we?

BODY & MIND

BODY & MIND

STEP 1 – PRACTICE MINDFULNESS MEDITATION

Mindfulness or mindfulness meditation is one of the most effective and highly recommended natural treatments for panic disorders. This technique is all about being aware of your present moment without making any judgments.

Through this technique, you can learn how to see things more clearly as well as being able to become more focused on your present situation. According to a study conducted by researchers at Lund University in Sweden, mindfulness is just as effective as cognitive behavioral therapy, which is all about replacing negative thinking patterns with positive ones.

In another study conducted at Boston University, researchers have found that mindfulness helps people with depression and anxiety let go of negative thoughts and stop obsessing over them. At the end of the study, the participants were able to get out of their depressive or anxious loop.

Furthermore, researchers have found that mindfulness meditation can help you sleep better, regulate mood levels, and alleviate stress, allowing you to relax and prevent panic attacks from occurring.

If you want your quality of life to improve, there is no doubt that mindfulness meditation can really be helpful and the beautiful part is;

It's so wonderfully easy to learn!

Why Mindfulness Meditation?

Mindfulness mediation sounds a bit airy-fairy. Yes. Of course it does. It conjures images of hippies or monks sitting on top of a mountain gently murmuring *"oooommmmm"* to themselves. Whilst that's not exactly the type of mediation we're talking about here, they seem like pretty chilled out guys right? Maybe they're on to something with the whole *meditation* thing.

What we're talking about is an incredible tool to tap into the present moment. Ultimately, what this helps you to do is see the symptoms you're having and view them *objectively*.

Why is this so important? Well, if you've ever experienced a panic attack, you can probably attest to the fact that, regardless of what starts it, when you're in the middle of it, you're only ever thinking about the worst situation and being about as far from objective as you can be.

"I'm having a heart attack, I'm going to die. OMG my family are going to be sad. What have I done with my life?" and so on.

What the practice of being mindful brings you is the ability to take a step back from the moment, look at the symptoms objectively and say;

"Ahhh, I see there's a bit of a tight chest feeling. That's OK. It doesn't mean I'm having a heart attack. It is what it is."

"I see that there are all these thoughts about how I feel I might be going insane. That's OK. I don't need to understand these thoughts, I just need to notice them for what they are."

"Looking at all these symptoms I can see that really, this is my body's reaction to something. My body is over-reacting because it thinks I am in danger. But I'm not. I will observe these symptoms until they pass and go about my day."

How to Practice Mindfulness Meditation

The short answer is:

Take a seat, pay attention to your breath, and when you notice your attention has wandered, return your attention to the breath.

For a slightly more in-depth run through:

- Find good posture with your back upright and relaxed in a chair or on a cushion. You can use a blanket and a pillow, although a good cushion that will last you a lifetime of practice. You can sit in a chair with your feet on the floor, loosely cross-legged, in lotus posture (if you're that flexible), kneeling etc. However you sit is fine, as long as you're comfortable. Just make sure you are stable and upright. If the constraints of your body prevent you from sitting erect, just find a comfortable position you can stay in for a while.
- Once you're sitting comfortably, start to feel your breath as it goes in and out. Really try to follow the breath all the way through your mouth, into your lungs, filling your belly, and then back out again.
- Inevitably, your attention will leave the breath and wander to other places. This happens to everyone.

It's literally part of the practice so don't stress about doing it wrong!
- When you do notice this, weather that's in a few seconds, a minute or five minutes, just return your attention to the breath. Don't worry about judging yourself or obsessing over the content of the thoughts.
- You focus. Your mind wanders. You notice this and re-focus on the breath, and repeat. That's the practice.

It's incredibly simple, but it's not necessarily easy. Just keep doing it and you'll get the results.

It's not as easy as saying *"I command myself to quit thinking of anything else besides my breath that I have decided to focus on."* Because you'll find yourself thinking about cat food or whatever. The point is that you *realize* you have strayed off course. Then you can gently bring your attention back to the breath and become present again.

Practice letting go of things you don't have control over. Oftentimes, people become anxious and experience panic attacks simply because they keep worrying about certain things happening or not happening.

For example; you can't control accidents, natural calamities, feelings of other people, and a whole host of other things. Remember that you're not a God (unless you are, in which case, nice to meet you Mr. God), you're a human being. You can't control everything, no matter how much you want to.

So when you get into an accident or when a loved one passes away, there is nothing else to do but to accept the fact and move on. Always try to see the positive side of the incident, however hard it might be at the time.

Say, you are currently going through a divorce. Instead of viewing it as a huge loss, you can view it as a chance for a new beginning.

When you start looking for and focusing on the positives of everything, you'll find more of them. If you naturally have more good and positive things in your life, doesn't it stand to reason that you'll be happier with less anxiety?

In addition, your blood pressure will normalize. Oftentimes, stress and anxiety causes blood pressure to rise. In order to bring it back to its normal level, you need to let your blood vessels dilate. You can help this by taking a few deep breaths and releasing tension.

Interestingly, anxiety does not only affect your mind, but it also affects your body. It can actually trigger numerous physical changes and symptoms. Excessive anxiety can trigger the fight or flight response of your system, causing your lymphatic nervous system to release the stress hormone cortisol. This, in turn, can raise your blood sugar levels and triglycerides.

It can also cause shortness of breath, dizziness, dry mouth, nausea, sweating, and panic attacks.

The real positive of this is, once you get your anxiety in check with these steps, you may find some potentially long-standing health issues are alleviated, or at least lessened. When you practice relaxation techniques you trigger your relaxation response, which is characterized by warm feelings and a silent mental alertness.

Cool, huh?

3

STEP 2 – PRACTICE BODY SCANNING

Body scan meditation is a popular practice for alleviating stress. If you have a panic disorder or suffer from any sort of anxiety, practicing this technique can really help you prevent panic attacks and alleviate any background worries. It is actually very similar to progressive muscle relaxation, except that it involves focusing on the sensations of your body parts rather than relaxing and tensing the muscles.

How to Practice Body Scan Meditation

Body Scan Meditation is kind of similar to the mindfulness meditation we just discussed in it's practice and application. You're doing something that brings you into the present moment.

Here's a great, in-depth run through of the steps for the awesome, StillMind:

1. Sit in a chair as for the breath awareness or lie down, making yourself comfortable, lying on your back on a mat or rug on the floor or on your bed. Choose a place where you will be warm and undisturbed. Allow your eyes to close gently.

2. Take a few moments to get in touch with the movement of your breath and the sensations in the body when you are ready, bring your awareness to the physical sensations in your body, especially to the sensations of touch or pressure, where your body makes contact with the chair or bed. On each outbreath, allow yourself to let go, to sink a little deeper into the chair or bed.

3. Remind yourself of the intention of this practice. Its aim is not to feel any different, relaxed, or calm; this may happen or it may not. Instead, the intention of the practice is, as best you can, to bring awareness to any sensations you detect, as you focus your attention on each part of the body in turn.

4. Now bring your awareness to the physical sensations in the lower abdomen, becoming aware of the changing patterns of sensations in the abdominal wall as you breathe in, and as you breathe out. Take a few minutes to feel the sensations as you breathe in and as you breathe out.

5. Having connected with the sensations in the abdomen, bring the focus or "spotlight" of your awareness down the left leg, into the left foot, and out to the toes of the left foot. Focus on each of the toes of the left foot in turn, bringing a gentle curiosity to investigate the quality of the sensations you find, perhaps noticing the sense of contact between the toes, a sense of tingling, warmth, or no particular sensation.

6. When you are ready, on an inbreath, feel or imagine the breath entering the lungs, and then passing down into the abdomen, into the left leg, the left foot, and out to the toes of the left foot. Then, on the outbreath, feel or imagine the breath coming all the way back up, out of the foot, into the leg, up through the abdomen, chest, and out through the nose. As best you can, continue this for a few breaths, breathing down into the toes, and back out from the toes. It may be difficult to get the hang of this just practice this "breathing into" as best you can, approaching it playfully.

7. Now, when you are ready, on an outbreath, let go of awareness of the toes, and bring your awareness to the sensations on the bottom of your left foot—bringing a gentle, investigative awareness to the sole of the foot, the instep, the heel (e.g., noticing the sensations where the heel makes contact with the mat or bed). Experiment with "breathing with" the sensations—being aware of the breath in the background, as, in the foreground, you explore the sensations of the lower foot.

8. Now allow the awareness to expand into the rest of the foot— to the ankle, the top of the foot, and right into the bones and joints. Then, taking a slightly deeper breath, directing it down into the whole of the left foot, and, as the breath lets go on the outbreath, let go of the left foot completely, allowing the focus of awareness to move into the lower left leg—the calf, shin, knee, and so on, in turn.

9. Continue to bring awareness, and a gentle curiosity, to the physical sensations in each part of the rest of the body in turn - to the upper left leg, the right toes, right foot, right leg, pelvic area, back, abdomen, chest, fingers, hands, arms, shoulders, neck, head, and face. In each area, as best you can, bring the same detailed level of awareness and gentle curiosity to the bodily sensations present. As you leave each major area, "breathe in" to it on the inbreath, and let go of that region on the outbreath.

10. When you become aware of tension, or of other intense sensations in a particular part of the body, you can "breathe in" to them—using the inbreath gently to bring awareness right into the sensations, and, as best you can, have a sense of their letting go, or releasing, on the outbreath.

11. The mind will inevitably wander away from the breath and the body from time to time. That is entirely normal. It is what minds do. When you notice it, gently acknowledge it, noticing where the mind has gone off to, and then gently return your attention to the part of the body you intended to focus on.

After you have "scanned" the whole body in this way, spend a few minutes being aware of a sense of the body as a whole, and of the breath flowing freely in and out of the body.

If you find yourself falling asleep, you might find it helpful to prop your head up with a pillow, open your eyes, or do the practice sitting up rather than lying down.

You can adjust the time spent in this practice by using larger chunks of your body to become aware of or spending a shorter or longer time with each part.

STEP 3 – PRACTICE ANCHORING

It's not always easy to control your nerves. You need sufficient skills. Just think of it this way; You've been asked to give a speech. This is something that you have always dreamt of doing. You know that if you do well, you'll probably get a raise, you'll be able to buy that nice house you've always wanted... However, you've got those telltale butterflies in your stomach.

So what can you do about this? What if there was a magic button you could press that would give you instant calm and confidence? Well guess what…

What is Anchoring?

In NLP (neuro linguistic programming), anchoring refers to the process of associating an emotional response with a trigger so that the response may be quickly and powerfully changed.

In our case, this means you can use anchoring to associate

a calm mental state with a simple internal trigger to help calm down and eliminate anxiety quickly.

You do this by anchoring states of mind so you can fire the anchor and establish the state instantly.

A brief history:

Anchoring is kind of like Pavlov's experiments with dogs. Pavlov sounded a bell as the animal was given food. The animals salivated when they saw the food. After doing this a few times, the bell and the food being shown together, the bell alone made the dogs salivate. Poor dogs.

Anchors are stimuli that call forth states of mind - thoughts and emotions. For example, touching a knuckle of the left hand could be an anchor. Some anchors are involuntary. So the smell of bread may take you back to your childhood. A tune may remind you of a loved one. A touch can bring back memories and the past states. These anchors work automatically and you may not be aware of the triggers.

Establishing an anchor means producing the stimuli (the anchor) when the desired state is experienced so that the desired state is pared to the anchor.

Anchors can be visual, auditory or kinesthetic and can be quick and easy install (just like a piece of software.)

Installing Anchors

It's quite a simple process and once it's done, you can use the anchor whenever you need that little boost of calmness.

1. Decide on the state you want to anchor. For example being calm and relaxed.
2. Choose an anchor (or anchors) that you wish to trigger the desired state.

3. Recall a memory or imagine a situation where you can experience the state. So recall or imagine a time when you experienced being really calm and relaxed. A lazy afternoon on a beach or a chilled evening with your friends watching TV for example.
4. Active the anchor or anchors when the experience is vivid and you are in the desired state.
5. Release the anchors when the experience begins to fade. If you keep applying the anchor when the experience is fading, then you will anchor a drop in calmness and relaxation!
6. Do something else - open your eyes ... count down from 10 to break state and distract yourself.
7. Repeat the steps several times, each time making the memory more vivid. This is not actually required when the anchor is established at the high point of the experience. However, you can strengthen the anchor by establishing it at the high point of several such experiences.
8. Apply the anchor and check that the required state occurs.
9. Future pace the situation where you want to experience the desired state. Fire the anchor to check that it creates a sufficiently resourced state.
10. Check the anchor the next day to ensure it is a permanent anchor.

Tips for anchoring

- The anchor (or anchors) should be fired in exactly

the same way every time you link them to the resourceful experience.
- Anchor at the high point of the experience containing the resourceful state.
- If you do not experience the state when future pacing and especially if you experience anxiety, then stop applying the anchor. (You will anchor the negative state!)
- There is a knowingness which makes anchoring work that is established by the unconscious mind.
- You can strengthen the anchor by repeating the above process over several days.
- If you are in a situation where you experience the desired state in reality, then you can reestablish the anchor to that situation.

Anchoring can be an incredibly powerful tool to help overcome anxiety in the moment. It's also really useful for any other state you could want to have on demand.

Want to feel more energized? *Make an anchor.*

Want to feel more in love? *Make an anchor.*

There's almost endless possibilities, but for the purposes of this book, just make one that makes you feel calm. If you have a panic attack and you've for a calm anchor set, it will bring you back to calmness in an instant and that's really what we want isn't it?

BREATHING

BREATHING

STEP 4 – PRACTICE SIMPLE BREATHING TECHNIQUES

Breathing techniques are highly effective in stress management and panic attack prevention. You can practice them whenever and wherever you are. So even if you can't get away from a stressful situation, you can still calm yourself down and prevent the onset of a panic attack.

These techniques let you experience relief from stress without going anywhere. You can stay at your desk and perform breathing exercises. You can do them while you're driving. You can do them while you're out with friends and in this way, you will always have a tool to use whenever you feel anxious and you can quickly and easily calm yourself.

Now you can try a million and one breathing exercises (and I suggest that you do). You can spend hours on YouTube and on blogs trying the different methods, but for me, one technique stands out above all the rest. It's so simple, so quick and so effective. I use it to calm me down if I'm having a panic attack or a feel one coming on. I use it to fall asleep. I use it to relax if I'm nervous about making a speech. I use it for anything and everything.

The 4 – 7 – 8 Exercise

If you only take away 1 thing from this book, **let it be this**.

This little technique has had the *biggest impact* for me in reducing my panic attacks.

"The 4-7-8 Breathing Exercise" also called *"The Relaxing Breath"* is based on pranayama, an ancient Indian practice that means *"regulation of breath."* The exercise is described by Dr. Andrew Weil as *"a natural tranquilizer for the nervous system"* that eases the body into a state of calmness and relaxation. Sounds good right?

There are different theories as to why it works so well but mainly the belief is that it encourages the fast removal of carbon dioxide from the body.

Dr. Weil's technique is beautifully simple, takes pretty much no time, and can be done anywhere in just five steps. Although you can do the exercise in any position, it's recommended to sit with your back straight while learning the exercise, kind of like the position we discussed for meditation.

Dr. Weil explains to "place the tip of your tongue against the ridge of tissue just behind your upper front teeth and keep it there through the entire exercise. You will be exhaling through your mouth around your tongue; try pursing your lips slightly if this seems awkward." This is followed by the five-step procedure listed below:

1. Exhale completely through your mouth, making a whoosh sound.
2. Close your mouth and inhale quietly through your nose to a mental count of four.

3. Hold your breath for a count of seven.
4. Exhale completely through your mouth, making a whoosh sound to a count of eight.
5. This is one breath. Now inhale again and repeat the cycle three more times for a total of four breaths.

Dr. Weil emphasizes the most important part of this process is holding your breath for eight seconds. This is because keeping the breath in will allow oxygen to fill your lungs and then circulate throughout the body. It is this that produces a relaxing effect in the body.

I've said it before and I'll say it again:

THIS ONE TECHNEQUE WILL RID YOU OF A PANIC ATTACK

If you feel one coming on or you're in the middle of one, just run through a couple of cycles of this breathing exercise and you'll be calm in no time!

STEP 5 – PRACTICE YOGIC BREATHING

Sometimes when your day becomes too stressful to handle, you may have a hard time sleeping at night. Some people have bedtime rituals, like; lighting a scented candle, writing in a journal, meditating, or drinking chamomile tea (I'm more of an English Breakfast tea kind of guy, but whatever floats your boat).

If meditation is not exactly your thing, you can still reap similar benefits without practicing it. Yoga incorporates a couple of breathing techniques that you may find to be useful.

Don't worry. I'm not going to ask you to fold yourself into any crazy yoga positions. I can't do any of that myself. What is laid out below is further breathing exercises that have been used for literally hundreds of years by the yogic community with some pretty solid results.

Alternate Nostril Breathing
This yogic breathing technique promotes deep relaxation

through the balance of the right and left sides of the brain as the nervous system is calmed down.

- **Sit down with both of your legs crossed or propped up on a pillow.** You can also kneel down next to the bed. Feel free to use blankets or any other object that can provide you with adequate support.
- **Rest your left hand over your left thigh.** The fingers on your right hand should be extended as if you are trying to wave at someone. Bend your middle and index fingers so that they curl inside your palm.
- **Put your thumb on the side of your nose and slightly touch your nostrils.** When you touch your nostrils, be careful not to be constricting. The idea is to limit airflow temporarily to one nostril.
- **Take a deep inhale and then exhale.** Close off your right nostril using your thumb. Breathe in through your left nostril for four seconds. When you reach the peak of that breath, you should close off your left nostril using your ring finger.
- **For four counts, hold this position to retain the breath.** Release your right nostril and breathe out for four seconds.
- **Then, take a deep breath for four seconds through your right nostril.** Just like what you did before, close it off, hold the position, and retain your breath for four seconds. Release your left nostril as you breathe out fully for four seconds.

Take a deep breath through your left nostril and repeat the entire cycle.

You can do this breathing technique as often as you want. When you're done, you can have a lie down on your bed and doze off or continue on with your day in a more relaxed state.

Deep Throat Breathing

This yoga breathing technique relaxes the body and calms the mind. You'll need to be in bed or on a comfortable floor for this one.

- **Simply lie down on your back with your legs wide apart.** Keep them as wide as your hips. Relax your arms at your sides and close your eyes.
- **Breathe in deeply through your nose and breathe out through your mouth.** With every breath you take, you should fill your lungs totally. Similarly, with every exhale you do, breathe out completely.
- **After taking three deep breaths,** inhale through your nose for four counts while constricting the back of your throat a bit. This way, you will feel as if you are breathing through a straw at the back of your throat as well as filling your lungs with air.
- **You should notice the sound of your breath mimicking the sound of waves that come in and out.** This sound is actually very helpful in making

you fall asleep. You can compare it to the soft snore of a baby.
- **Hold your breath at the top for four seconds as you silently observe your feelings.** You should aim to feel relaxed and full. Breathe out through your nose for four seconds while constricting your throat a little.
- Once your lungs have released all the air, you should begin to fill them again.
- Take a deep breath for six seconds and hold it for another six seconds.
- Finally, breathe out for six seconds.
- Repeat this breathing process, adding two seconds more for every cycle.

After you reached your maximum capacity of breathing and holding, you can begin taking away a couple of seconds at a time. So, if twelve seconds is the maximum amount of time that you can do, your next round should be down to ten seconds. Continue subtracting two seconds every time, so the next round is eight seconds, and so on.

When you reach four seconds, you can release everything and return to normal breathing. Now that you have relaxed your mind and body, you can have a peaceful sleep and wake up feeling refreshed and rejuvenated.

DIET

DIET

WHAT YOU EAT EFFECTS YOUR BRAIN

"You are what you eat."

We've all heard it. It's usually a well-meant comment from someone trying to steer you away from chips and a burger toward something a bit more green and healthy.

I used to dismiss this, especially in my younger years. I thought I could eat what I wanted (usually a big bowl of pasta) and be fine. And that *was* the case…for a while.

At some point or another in my late teens, I lost my job. At the time this was the best thing that had ever happened to me.

"So you're saying I can go to bed when I want, sleep for 13 hours, get up when I want and basically spend my days doing nothing and chilling?...Sign me up, that sounds awesome!"

That was pretty much the attitude. A lot's changed since then and I am not the same person I was. I'm up early every day improving myself and working towards big goals, but at the time, this lazy mentality made sense to me.

The point is, at the time I got into a routine of sleeping a lot, waking up, eating a big bowl of pasta and cheese (similar to mac & cheese for our American friends, just without the lovely baked finish) and then feeling tired, zoned out and uninspired for the rest of the day.

I was sleeping for 12-13 hours a day and I was still tired all the time. What's that about?

Unsurprisingly, this *"life without any goals"* happened to be around the time anxiety & depression first visited me. Coincidence? I think not.

I found a stark change in my energy and anxiety came when I found a job and started eating "better" at work. My anxiety went. My depression went. I was happier *because* I was healthier.

As you can probably guess by the title of the chapter, my opinion on the matter is pretty resolute:

WHAT YOU EAT AFFECTS YOUR MOOD

There are so many studies on how gut bacteria affect your mood and there are so many studies on how different foods effect how you feel.

As a simple example;

Have you ever eaten lunch?...I thought so. Now, have you ever eaten a *BIG* lunch? I'm talking a couple of sandwiches, maybe some pasta, a fizzy drink and a chocolate or doughnut to finish it off?

Now tell me, how did you feel about an hour after that?

Did you feel like you were about to fall asleep and you couldn't think quite as clearly as before? Did you feel a bit slow and lethargic for the rest of the day? Most likely. If not, you're some sort of medical anomaly and you could make good money selling your body to science.

This is just a really simple illustration as to how food can immediately affect your mind and physiology.

It's not too much of a stretch then, if this extra bit of sugar at lunch can affect you so drastically, that eating a sub-optimal diet can contribute to other things over the long term, namely, anxiety and panic attacks.

We already know that excess carbohydrates cause obesity (don't worry, this isn't turning into a diet book). With the global rise in obesity, we're seeing a strong correlation with a rise in neuro-degenerative diseases such as Alzheimer's which a number of scientists have called to be re-labeled Type 3 diabetes as it results from resistance to insulin in the brain.

What science is saying then, is that excess carbohydrates, in vast quantities over a period of years, can cause serious damage in the body and mind.

BUT...

The good news is; there is *always* something you can do about it.

The answer seems to be eating a lower carbohydrate and a higher, healthy fat diet.

Why you ask?

We're starting to see strong evidence for healthy fats improving cognitive function in patients with Alzheimer's.

If that sentence alone doesn't excite you, the same concept is being applied in other areas of medicine and there's a lot of scientists getting really excited about the fact that a low carb, high fat (ketogenic) diet seems to have some pretty profound effect on inflammation in the body and a whole heap of other stuff.

I tried going on a ketogenic diet for 30 days. And I had…0 panic attacks. I started eating carbs again and they started to come back.

I've also experimented with eliminating caffeine (well, coffee anyway, I'm British so there's no way I'm not going to drink tea) and have had some pretty profound results with it.

No more caffeine = No more anxiety*

*For me at least!

Now I don't want this chapter to be a pitch for a low-carb lifestyle, you'll find endless books and blogs proclaiming it to be the best thing since sliced bread (pun intended). What I wanted to show you was that what you eat can really effect how you feel and preform.

So when I say; *Try giving up caffeine for 30 days and watch your anxiety lessen...*

I know it works, and this chapter is about showing you that.

What you put into your body makes a big difference on your anxiety and panic response also.

So, eat better and feel better because of it!

NEXT STEPS

NEXT STEPS

QUICK START GUIDE

So this is all well and good. But how do you actually implement any of this?

Well, let's keep it simple;

1. Try the 4/7/8 breathing method whenever you feel a panic attack coming on and any other time you want to just relax…Try it now…go on, I'll wait.
2. Cut out caffeine (just for 30 days) – You can get back to your double, triple mocha late crap after a month if you feel it hasn't made a difference
3. Start practicing mindfulness meditation daily – It only needs to take 10 minutes. If you only had to spend 10 minutes a day on something and it eliminated your anxiety and panic attacks, would you do it? Exactly, that's what I thought.

The idea with any of the techniques in the book is to practice them at a time when you don't need them, so you can easily call upon them when you do need them.

Most of these can be performed anywhere, any time and without anyone really noticing. Even if you have to excuse yourself for a minute or two and run through a couple of deep breathing cycles in the restroom, it's not quite as much of an inconvenience as having a panic attack whilst at your desk at work!

So get practicing and you'll find your anxiety begins to lessen and lessen further until you can really live your life to the fullest!

You always have choices and choosing to eliminate anxiety seems like a pretty sound one.

AFTERWORD

Panic attacks can be a horrible experience for anyone but, given the right tools and techniques, anyone can overcome them and live a full life.

The methods outlined in this book will help you to take charge again so, if you ever feel another attack coming on, you have everything you need to regain control again, quickly.

You've now got the tools to work towards lessening the frequency of the attacks until they're just a distant memory.

You can do it. It's not even that difficult. If you truly want to change and rid yourself of panic attacks, the steps outlined in this book will get you there.

Now go out there and live your life on your terms!!!

UNTITLED

Thank You

Thank you again for downloading this book!

I hope this book was able to help you to eliminate panic attacks and regain control of your life.

The next step is to go out there and live your life to the fullest!

Finally, if you enjoyed this book, then I'd like to ask you for a favor, would you be kind enough to leave a review for this book on Amazon? It'd be greatly appreciated!

Thank you and good luck!

Ed Jones

www.ingramcontent.com/pod-product-compliance
Lightning Source LLC
Chambersburg PA
CBHW060413080526
44583CB00012B/553